THE PLANT PARADOX LIFESTYLE

18 Steps to Help You Lose Weight, Reduce Chronic Inflammation, Heal Your Gut and Rapidly Improve Your Health

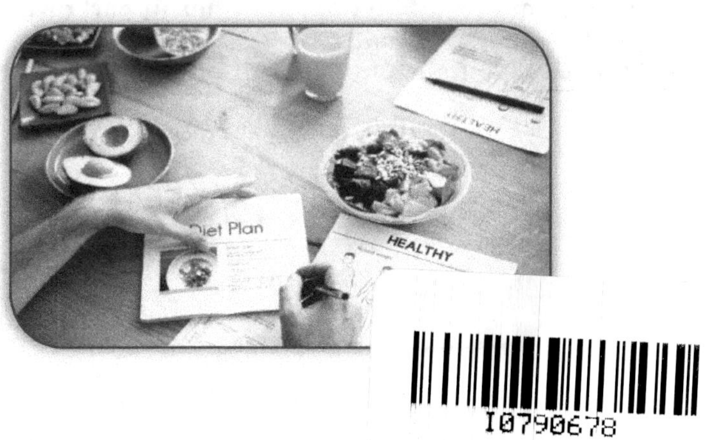

NATHALIE SMITH

Copyright © 2024 by Nathalie Smith

Disclaimer:

This book is intended for educational purposes only and provides an overview of health theories outlined by various health professionals, along with insights into how I implemented them in my own journey. Please keep in mind that every single individual is distinct, therefore what suits one person might not suit another. For personalized medical advice, diagnosis, or treatment, always consult with your doctor or a qualified healthcare professional.

TABLE OF CONTENT

INTRODUCTION

How I Transformed My Health with the Plant Paradox Program: A Personal Journey

If you're feeling overwhelmed by the flood of information about healthy living, I get it. That was me a few years ago before I discovered the Plant Paradox program. Like many of you, I was trying to eat right, stay active, and take care of my body, but despite my best efforts, my health was deteriorating. This is my story of how I regained control over my health by adopting the Plant Paradox lifestyle.

My Health Struggles Before the Plant Paradox

In my late 30s, I began experiencing a range of health issues that left me puzzled. Despite eating what I believed to be a healthy diet and getting frequent exercise, I was gaining weight. I struggled with daily acid reflux that was so severe I couldn't fall asleep lying down. My PMS symptoms and cramps were unbearable, and I had a host of other issues like inexplicable acne, dry skin, and hair loss. I was constantly fatigued, needing naps after my morning yoga sessions, and my body felt stiff and achy all the time.

These symptoms, which are often dismissed as "normal" for women approaching their 40s, were becoming too much for me to handle. I couldn't accept that my health was destined to decline, so I started searching for answers.

The Turning Point: Discovering the Plant Paradox

One day, while scrolling through my Facebook feed, I stumbled upon an article titled "Are We Wrong About What Makes Food Healthy?" It was an interview with

Dr. Steven Gundry, and it was the first time I heard the term "lectins." The article made me realize that the foods I thought were healthy might have been contributing to my health problems.

My Pre-Plant Paradox Lifestyle

Before adopting the Plant Paradox program, my diet looked like this:

- **Breakfast:** Organic oats with non-dairy milk, goji berries, and banana slices, or whole wheat bread with peanut butter and berries.

- **Lunch:** A platter with green salad, tomatoes, cucumbers, bell peppers, feta cheese, hummus, olives, and whole wheat bread.

- **Dinner:** Often out at restaurants, but I made "healthy" choices like avoiding the bun on a burger, opting for sweet potato fries, and sharing meals with my husband.

- Grocery Shopping: I always chose grass-fed meat, wild-caught fish, and pastured chicken and eggs. I rarely drank soda and only indulged in fast food once a month.

Despite these efforts, I found myself constantly buying new clothes because nothing fit anymore. I avoided the scale out of fear, but when I finally weighed myself, I was horrified to see I was 22 pounds heavier than my normal weight. This was a wake-up call, and I knew I had to make a change.

Making Up My Mind to Get Healthy

One of the most important things I've learned is that getting healthy is within our power, but it requires a firm decision to change. As someone once told me, *"You won't make a change until you're fed up with being fed up."* That was exactly my situation, and it pushed me to explore new ways to improve my health.

The Impact of the Plant Paradox on My Health

Since starting the Plant Paradox program in August 2017, all my health issues have been resolved. I've lost the extra fat and water, built muscle, and improved my metabolism. My periods are now easy, my body is no longer stiff, and I don't experience midday crashes.

Sinus headaches, which used to be a constant problem, are now rare, and I've managed them with natural remedies like turmeric, ginger, and elderberry syrup instead of relying on medication.

Beyond the Plant Paradox: Expanding My Knowledge

While Dr. Gundry's book provided many answers, I was eager to learn more. I started following other health experts whose advice aligned with the Plant Paradox principles. What I've realized is that while many diet theories share common principles, the lectin-free lifestyle, in particular, has been a game-changer for those dealing with chronic inflammation.

The Plant Paradox as a Lifestyle, Not a Diet

One of the key things I've learned is that the Plant Paradox isn't just a diet; it's a lifestyle. I'm so grateful for the health transformation I've experienced that I've made it my mission to share this information with others. I believe that making these dietary and lifestyle changes sustainable is key to long-term success, and cooking and enjoying good food is a big part of that.

Before You Start: Understanding the Bigger Picture

It's important to understand how we got here and to shift our perspective on healing, medicine, and food. While weight gain is often the first symptom that motivates us to change, it's not the only indicator of health issues. I encourage you to seek health, not just weight loss, as your ultimate goal. Once you remove the factors causing inflammation and pain, your body will naturally restore its balance.

Adopting the Plant Paradox lifestyle has been a transformative journey for me. It has allowed me to regain control of my health and well-being in ways I never thought possible. While it may seem overwhelming at first, the benefits far outweigh the challenges. If you're struggling with similar health issues, I encourage you to explore this lifestyle and see the difference it can make in your life.

CHAPTER 1

The 18 Essential Steps to Transform Your Health with the Plant Paradox Lifestyle

Step 1: Dig Yourself Out of the Omega-6 Hole

One of the most critical steps to reducing chronic inflammation and improving your health is cutting down on Omega-6 fatty acids. These fats, found in industrial seed oils like canola, sunflower, and grapeseed oil, are often marketed as "heart healthy," but in reality, they're highly inflammatory. To support your body, replace these oils with healthier options such as extra virgin olive oil, avocado oil, coconut oil, grass-fed ghee, or perilla oil. Additionally, removing highly processed foods, as highlighted in Step 5, is essential for balancing your Omega-3 to Omega-6 ratio.

It's shocking how widespread these harmful oils are; just read the labels at the supermarket. You'll find them in everything from salad dressings and mayonnaise to margarine, imitation butters, and even baked goods like cookies and cakes. These oils are hidden in many everyday items, contributing to inflammation without us even realizing it.

When I first moved to the US, I fell into the trap of buying vegan butter, grapeseed oil, and canola oil, believing the "heart-healthy" claims on the packaging. I thought I was making smart choices, but I was misled by the overwhelming amount of false health information. My health began to decline until I discovered the Plant Paradox program, which helped me understand the true impact of these oils on my body.

Step 2: Remove Grains and Soy from Your Diet

Eliminating grains and soy from your diet is a powerful move toward better health. While it might seem daunting to give up bread, pizza, and pasta, you'll be pleasantly surprised to discover delicious alternatives that allow you to enjoy these foods in moderation without relying on wheat or corn.

If you absolutely must keep one grain in your diet, opt for real sourdough bread made with only salt, organic flour, water, and a sourdough starter. Treat it as a weekend indulgence, perfect for soaking up extra virgin olive oil.

As for soy sauce, which is a staple in many kitchens, there are excellent replacements available. Coconut aminos and high-quality fermented soy sauces, like Japanese umami, offer great flavor without the negative effects of traditional soy products.

Research has shown that inflammation is the root of many degenerative conditions, including brain disorders. Gluten and high-carbohydrate diets are significant triggers of inflammatory pathways that can affect the brain.

Grains, often considered healthy due to their vitamin and fiber content, can spike blood sugar just as effectively as table sugar. The starches in grains break down into glucose as soon as you start chewing, leading to blood sugar spikes and contributing to inflammation.

By removing grains and soy from your diet, you can reduce inflammation and improve your overall health, while still enjoying satisfying and delicious meals.

Step 3: Cut Sugar from Your Diet

Sugar is not just a treat; it's an addictive substance that plays a significant role in modern chronic illnesses. From insulin resistance to non-alcoholic fatty liver disease and kidney disease, sugar consumption is at the root of many health problems we face today.

Whether it's refined sugar, corn syrup, agave syrup, maple syrup, or even honey, all these sweeteners have a similar impact on your insulin levels. They disrupt your gut health and cause damage to your cells.

While there are alternative sweeteners like inulin, erythritol, and monk fruit that are generally considered safe, it's important to use them sparingly. The sweet taste itself can be addictive, and regular consumption of these substitutes can lead to increased cravings, which is something you want to avoid.

Re-educating your palate to not crave sweetness is key. By reducing your dependence on sugary foods, you can improve your health and reduce the risk of chronic diseases. If you're craving something sweet, dark chocolate with 1g or less of sugar per serving is a good option in moderation.

The problem with sweetness, whether from sugar or calorie-free substitutes, is that your body can't distinguish between them. Your brain expects calories when it tastes sweetness, and when they don't arrive, it drives you to seek out more sweet foods. This cycle can lead to overeating and continued cravings, undermining your health goals.

Breaking free from sugar's grip is essential to improving your overall health and well-being.

Step 4: Treat Fruit Like Candy

It might be surprising, but treating fruit like candy is a crucial step in managing your sugar intake. Except for avocados, lemons, and limes, most fruits are high in natural sugars, and consuming them in large quantities can spike your blood sugar levels just like candy does. Our ancestors didn't have access to the abundance of fruit we do today, and our bodies haven't evolved to handle this much sugar from fruit.

While you don't need to eliminate fruit entirely, moderation is key. Focus on enjoying fruits that are in season and locally ripened, as they are often fresher and have lower sugar content. Berries are an excellent choice because they are lower in sugar compared to other fruits and are packed with antioxidants.

Think of fruit as an occasional treat rather than a staple of your diet. By limiting your intake and choosing lower-sugar options, you can enjoy the benefits of fruit without overloading your system with sugar. This approach helps manage blood sugar levels and supports overall health.

Incorporate fruits mindfully into your meals. For example, add a small handful of berries to your morning yogurt or use a slice of lemon to flavor your water. This way, you can still enjoy the flavor and nutrients of fruit without the sugar overload. By treating fruit like a special treat rather than an everyday staple, you'll maintain better control over your sugar intake and improve your overall health.

Step 5: Eat REAL FOOD or Remove All Highly Processed Food

Eating real food and cutting out highly processed foods is essential for reducing inflammation, improving health, and maintaining a healthy weight. Processed foods are often loaded with hidden sugars, unhealthy fats, and artificial ingredients that can wreak havoc on your body. Most of these foods come in packages and are designed to be convenient but at the cost of your health.

Highly processed foods are typically made with inflammatory oils like corn, soybean, and cottonseed oil, which contribute to chronic inflammation and various health issues. These foods also contain preservatives, additives, and artificial flavors that can harm your gut health and disrupt your body's natural processes.

To protect your health, it's crucial to become a label reader. When shopping for groceries, take the time to examine the ingredients list on packaged foods. If you see a long list of ingredients you can't pronounce, or if sugar and unhealthy oils are listed, it's best to put that item back on the shelf. Instead, focus on buying whole, unprocessed foods that are close to their natural state, such as fresh vegetables, fruits, nuts, seeds, and high-quality proteins.

By avoiding processed foods and choosing real, whole foods, you'll not only reduce your intake of harmful substances but also increase your consumption of nutrients that support overall health.

This shift can lead to improved energy levels, better digestion, and even weight loss. Remember, eating real food isn't just about avoiding the bad stuff; it's about nourishing your body with the best possible fuel.

Step 6: Reduce Animal Protein Consumption and Choose the Best Quality

When it comes to animal protein, quality matters as much as quantity. It's not just about what you eat; it's about what the animal you're eating was fed.

Opting for high-quality protein means choosing meat from animals raised in their natural environments, grazing on grass, and living in open pastures.

Look for labels like "100% grass-fed" or "grass-fed, grass-finished" when selecting beef, and choose wild-caught, sustainable fish and shellfish whenever possible.

While protein is essential for health, we often consume more than necessary. Many experts now agree that the amount of protein most of us have been told to eat is excessive.

In fact, we can meet a significant portion of our protein needs from plant-based sources. A good rule of thumb for portion size is to use the palm of your hand (excluding fingers) as a guide—anything larger is likely too much.

One concept that embodies this approach is "condimeat," where animal protein is used as a condiment rather than the main ingredient of a meal. This idea aligns with a growing movement known as the "pagan" lifestyle, popularized by Dr. Mark Hyman, which combines the best aspects of both paleo and vegan diets.

The focus is on making vegetables the centerpiece of your meals, with small amounts of high-quality animal protein as an accompaniment.

This step is a key principle of the plant paradox lifestyle, which encourages us to rethink our relationship with animal protein, emphasizing quality over quantity, and promoting a diet rich in plant-based food.

Step 7: Eliminate Nightshades and Legumes Temporarily or Prepare Them Properly

As someone who once adored tomatoes, bell peppers, and cucumbers, I understand how surprising and difficult it might be to hear that these seemingly healthy vegetables can be problematic.

While they do offer some nutrients (and let's not forget that some are technically fruits), they are also packed with anti-nutrients like lectins, which can cause significant inflammation for some people.

If you can't imagine life without nightshades, there are ways to make them safer to eat. Peel and deseed them; this is where most of the lectins reside. As for legumes, they are notorious for their high anti-nutrient content and can be tough on digestion.

Most cases of food poisoning worldwide are due to undercooked beans. Try cutting out legumes for a while to give your gut time to heal. If you find it challenging to eliminate them, especially if you follow a vegetarian diet, you can gradually reintroduce them later, but always ensure they are pressure-cooked to reduce their lectin content.

Personally, after following this approach and healing my gut, I was able to reintroduce both nightshades and legumes into my diet but only when prepared properly.

A traditional Romanian dish made from tomatoes, peppers, and eggplant became a go-to meal once I modified the recipe to lower its lectin content. This shows that some foods don't need to be banned forever; with the right preparation, they can be enjoyed again.

So, what exactly are lectins? In essence, lectins are large proteins found in plants and animals that serve as a defense mechanism for plants. They attach to sugar molecules in our bodies, leading to potential disruptions in cellular communication and triggering toxic or inflammatory responses.

This binding process is why lectins are sometimes called "sticky proteins," as they can interfere with various bodily functions, especially in the gut and other sensitive areas.

Step 8: Understand Your Nuts and Seeds

Nuts can be a fantastic addition to your diet when consumed in moderation. However, it's crucial to understand that not everything labeled as a nut is actually a nut. Peanuts and cashews, for example, are not true nuts and are highly inflammatory. This distinction is important for anyone looking to reduce inflammation and improve overall health.

When it comes to almonds, you should be aware that their skins are packed with anti-nutrients, particularly lectins. To avoid these, opt for blanched almonds, which have had their skins removed, making them a much safer and healthier choice.

Seeds are another area where knowledge is key. While sunflower, pumpkin, and chia seeds are popular, they are also rich in lectins. If you're looking to reduce inflammation, consider choosing less inflammatory options like hemp, flax, and sesame seeds. These seeds are not only lower in lectins but also provide a host of beneficial nutrients without the potential downsides.

By understanding the differences between nuts and seeds, and making informed choices about which to include in your diet, you can enjoy their benefits while minimizing any negative impacts.

Step 9: Not All Dairy Is Created Equal

First, it's important to understand that dairy milk, regardless of its source, is loaded with sugar and insulin-like growth hormones designed to promote rapid growth in calves. For those looking to reduce sugar intake and avoid these growth hormones, dairy milk might not be the best choice.

Thankfully, there are numerous delicious and healthy alternatives like hemp, almond, and macadamia milk, which can even be made at home with ease. Hemp milk, in particular, is a great non-dairy option, and making it yourself ensures you know exactly what's in it.

Another crucial aspect to consider is the type of casein protein in dairy products. Cows worldwide can be classified into two categories based on the type of casein they produce: A1 and A2. Most cattle in North America and Northern Europe produce casein A1, which has been linked to various health issues.

In contrast, cattle from Southern Europe primarily produce casein A2, which is generally considered a healthier option. If you wish to keep dairy in your diet, opt for French, Swiss, or Italian-aged cheeses and butter, but in moderation.

Goat and sheep dairy products are also safer alternatives to cow's milk. However, like all dairy, treating them as condiments rather than the main ingredient in your meals is best. In my personal experience, I've found that dairy doesn't agree with me, so I've largely eliminated it, except for the occasional small serving of butter.

Understanding the difference between casein A1 and A2, as well as the impact of dairy on your health, allows you to make more informed choices that align with the Plant Paradox lifestyle.

Step 10: Make Vegetables and High-Quality Fats the Core of Your Diet

When you first eliminate nightshades and legumes from your diet, you might feel like your food options have suddenly shrunk. I felt the same way, especially since these foods are often front and center in supermarkets and have long been staples in many diets.

However, once you shift your focus, you'll discover a whole new world of delicious, nutrient-dense foods that are far healthier for you.

Start by embracing green leafy vegetables like Swiss chard, kale, mustard greens, spinach, and collard greens. These are packed with nutrients and should be a staple on your plate.

Then, explore the world of cruciferous vegetables such as cauliflower, broccoli, cabbage, and Brussels sprouts. These vegetables not only offer a wealth of health benefits but are also incredibly versatile in cooking.

Don't forget about other nutritious options like asparagus, celery, carrots, artichokes, and root vegetables like parsnips, rutabaga, turnips, and various types of sweet potatoes and yams.

Salad greens, including romaine, butter lettuce, and radicchio, can also be delicious additions to your meals.

Herbs and microgreens, particularly broccoli microgreens, are excellent for adding a nutritional boost to dishes or even smoothies.

Making these vegetables a regular part of your diet will not only enhance your health but also broaden your culinary horizons. Incorporating high-quality fats, such as avocados, extra virgin olive oil, and coconut or MCT oils, will further support your health journey. These fats are essential for absorbing fat-soluble vitamins and supporting overall well-being.

Once you move beyond nightshades and legumes, you'll find that there's an abundance of healthy, satisfying options that will keep you nourished and energized.

Step 11: Consume fermented foods

Incorporating fermented foods into your daily diet is a centuries-old practice that has been recognized for its health advantages across cultures.

Fermentation not only preserves food but also increases its nutritional value, making it an important part of a balanced diet.

Fermented foods contain probiotics, which are beneficial bacteria that assist in maintaining a healthy gut microbiome. A healthy gut is essential for general well-being since it regulates digestion, immunological function, and even mental health.

Consuming fermented foods on a daily basis can help to promote the growth of these beneficial gut bacteria, which are essential for maintaining your digestive system in top condition.

Yogurt, kefir, sauerkraut, kimchi, miso, tempeh, and kombucha are all great fermented food options. These foods are not only delicious, but they also provide a range of flavors and textures to complement your meals.

Make it a habit to incorporate at least one serving of fermented food into your daily diet. Whether it's a teaspoon of sauerkraut with lunch, a glass of kefir in the morning, or some miso soup for dinner, these foods are simple to incorporate into your daily routine.

Your gut health will improve over time, resulting in better digestion, a stronger immune system, and overall vitality. Eating fermented foods daily is a simple yet effective strategy to improve your overall health.

Step 12: Balance Feeding with Fasting

Balancing feeding with fasting is not about depriving yourself but finding a rhythm that supports your body's natural cycles. When you follow the previous steps, you'll notice a significant reduction in hunger pangs and cravings. You can enjoy nutrient-dense foods that nourish your gut without the need to count calories or constantly snack.

Intermittent fasting has been shown to offer numerous health benefits, including improved metabolism, enhanced brain function, and increased longevity.

By giving your body regular breaks from eating, you allow it to repair and rejuvenate, promoting overall wellness.

This approach leads to what I like to call "food freedom." You'll no longer feel controlled by hunger or tempted by unhealthy foods. Instead, you'll start craving wholesome, nourishing options like broccoli, avocados, eggs, and dark chocolate. You'll find yourself at ease, even when surrounded by less healthy choices, focusing on foods that truly make your body thrive.

I practice intermittent fasting by eating my final meal at 7 p.m. and not eating again until midday the next day. Initially, this routine took some adjustment, but now I find I simply don't need or want food in the morning.

Intermittent fasting helps you develop what Dr. Steven Gundry describes as "metabolic flexibility" in your mitochondria, the energy powerhouses of your cells, especially in your brain. This flexibility is crucial for long-term health and vitality.

Fasting is a practice rooted in tradition across various cultures and religions, not as a punishment but as a path to wellness. It's about giving your body the space to heal and flourish.

If you're ready to explore this further, consider trying a five-day fasting-mimicking diet meal plan that aligns with the principles of the Plant Paradox. This plan focuses on plant-based foods, avoiding animal proteins, and incorporating pressure-cooked beans, making it easier to support your health while practicing fasting.

Step 13: Supplement

We all have different nutritional requirements, and we should preferably undergo tests to determine what our bodies may be lacking. However, there are a few generic supplements that the majority of individuals can benefit from. These include DHA and EPA (high-quality fish or krill oil), magnesium and potassium, Vitamin D3 and K2, polyphenols, and vital vitamins and minerals such as biotin, selenium, and pro- and pre-biotics.

While I do not recommend that you start taking these supplements right now, you should do the necessary research. Consider seeing a functional medicine practitioner, taking pertinent tests, and deciding what's best for your body.

In a perfect world, supplementing would be unnecessary. Ideally, we would acquire all of the nutrients we require from our diet and surroundings. However, contemporary agricultural practices have drastically depleted the soil of key nutrients, and our increasingly detached lifestyles make it difficult to meet all of our needs through food alone.

Supplements can help cover these gaps, thereby improving your health and well-being. They should, however, be carefully selected and used to supplement, rather than replace, a well-balanced diet rich in whole, nutrient-dense foods.

Step 14: Use Quality Iodized Salt in Your Cooking

Contrary to what you may have heard for years, salt is not something to fear, especially when you choose the right kind. While many iodized sea salts on the market contain additives like dextrose, opting for pure, quality salt can make a big difference in your health.

Himalayan pink salt is an excellent choice, as it's naturally rich in minerals and iodine, providing the benefits of traditional iodized salt without unnecessary additives. It's important to ensure you're getting enough iodine in your diet, as it supports thyroid function and overall health.

For those looking for other high-quality salt options, you can explore various natural salts that are free from harmful additives. Remember, salt is essential for your body, so don't shy away from it. Just make sure you're using the best quality available to enhance your meals and support your well-being.

Step 15: Re-Learn the Pleasure and Art of Cooking

This step is intentionally placed near the end to emphasize that mastering the previous steps becomes much easier when you embrace cooking at home. To make this lifestyle sustainable, it's essential to find joy in preparing delicious, healthy meals for yourself and your loved ones or even cooking together.

The key is to enjoy the food you create more than anything you might order at a restaurant. When you reach that point, sticking to this lifestyle becomes second nature.

Cooking at home allows you to control what goes into your food, ensuring that you're consuming the healthiest ingredients possible. It's not just about nourishment but also about developing a deeper appreciation for the process of creating something that benefits your body and brings joy to your taste buds.

Unless you have the luxury of a private chef, rediscovering the pleasure of cooking is vital. It's often said that obesity and other health issues run in families, but more than genetics, it's the dietary and lifestyle habits that are passed down. By re-learning the art of cooking, you can break unhealthy cycles and create a legacy of health for yourself and your family.

Step 16: Try to Reduce Your Stress and Have Quality Sleep

This step is non-negotiable. Stress and poor-quality sleep can significantly harm both your body and mind. The good news is that making changes to your diet often leads to improvements in these areas, but it's crucial to actively assess and address your stress levels and sleep quality.

When we are stressed or sleep-deprived, our bodies struggle to function optimally. Chronic stress can lead to a host of health issues, including inflammation, weakened immunity, and mental health challenges. Similarly, lack of sleep affects cognitive functions, mood regulation, and even our ability to make sound decisions.

Research shows that sleep deprivation particularly affects the prefrontal cortex, the area of the brain responsible for planning, decision-making, and self-awareness. When we don't get enough sleep, this region becomes impaired, making it harder to regulate emotions and respond to situations rationally. Instead, the amygdala, the brain's "fear center," takes over, leading to increased anxiety and stress responses.

To truly thrive, it's essential to incorporate stress-reduction techniques, such as meditation, deep breathing exercises, or regular physical activity into your routine. Prioritizing quality sleep is also vital; aim for 7-9 hours per night. By focusing on these factors, you lay the groundwork for increased health, mood, and overall well-being.

Step 17: Assess and Address Exposure to "Deadly Disruptors"

To truly optimize your health, it's crucial to recognize and minimize exposure to various "deadly disruptors" that contribute to chronic inflammation. These disruptors are pervasive in our modern environment, and while it's challenging to avoid them entirely, being aware of their presence and taking proactive steps can significantly impact your well-being.

Common Disruptors Include:

1. Broad-Spectrum Antibiotics: While necessary at times, overuse can disrupt your gut microbiome, leading to inflammation and other health issues.

2. NSAIDs (Non-Steroidal Anti-Inflammatory Drugs): Medications like ibuprofen can harm the gut lining and contribute to inflammation when used frequently.

3. Stomach Acid Blockers: These can interfere with digestion and nutrient absorption, potentially leading to gut health problems.

4. Artificial Sweeteners: Substances like sucralose and aspartame are linked to metabolic disruptions and increased inflammation.

5. Endocrine Disruptors: Found in many household, skincare, and beauty products, these chemicals can interfere with hormone function and contribute to long-term health issues.

6. Environmental Toxins: Air pollution, mold exposure, arsenic in food, heavy metals, and plastic exposure are all linked to inflammation and various chronic diseases.

7. GMO Foods and Herbicides: Genetically modified organisms (GMOs) and chemicals like Roundup can disrupt gut health and promote inflammation.

8. Constant Exposure to Blue Light: Prolonged exposure to blue light from screens can interfere with sleep patterns, contributing to stress and inflammation.

Action Steps:

- Evaluate your environment and lifestyle for these disruptors.

- Opt for natural or organic products whenever possible, especially in skincare, household cleaning, and food choices.

- Limit the use of NSAIDs and artificial sweeteners, and consult with a healthcare professional about safer alternatives.

- Reduce screen time, especially before bed, and consider using blue light filters on your devices.

- Prioritize detoxifying practices such as drinking plenty of water, using air purifiers, and consuming a diet rich in antioxidants.

By being mindful of these disruptors and taking steps to minimize your exposure, you can reduce chronic inflammation and protect your long-term health.

Step 18: Keep Your Brain and Body Active

Staying active, both mentally and physically, is essential for overall well-being. Regular movement and mental stimulation help keep your brain sharp and your body strong, promoting longevity and a better quality of life.

- Physical Activity: Engaging in moderate exercise is crucial for maintaining a healthy body. Whether it's walking, jogging, yoga, or playing your favorite sport, find something you enjoy and make it a regular part of your routine.

Walking is one of the easiest and most effective ways to stay active. Try to choose it whenever possible, like taking the stairs instead of the elevator or going for a walk during your lunch break.

- **Mental Stimulation:** Keeping your brain active is just as important as physical exercise. Challenge yourself to learn new things regularly; whether it's picking up a new hobby, reading, or playing brain games like puzzles or strategy games. This not only keeps your mind sharp but also enhances cognitive function and mental resilience.

- **Mindfulness and Meditation:** Incorporating mindfulness practices like meditation into your routine can significantly reduce stress and improve mental clarity. Even a few minutes a day can help calm your mind, enhance focus, and contribute to emotional well-being.

- **Balance and Enjoyment:** The key is to find activities you genuinely enjoy, so that staying active feels less like a chore and more like a rewarding part of your day. Whether it's a morning walk, an evening game of tennis, or a quiet moment of meditation, these practices will keep both your body and mind in peak condition.

CHAPTER 2

Kelly Clarkson's Transformative Weight Loss Success Story

Kelly Clarkson's weight loss success story demonstrates the impact of long-term changes in lifestyle. For years, the singer struggled with weight shifts and health conditions such as thyroid disease and polycystic ovarian syndrome (PCOS). Despite her hectic schedule, Clarkson realized she needed to make a change.

Clarkson first learned about the Plant Paradox diet in 2018. This groundbreaking method focuses on avoiding lectin-containing foods, which can cause inflammation and discomfort in certain people. By following this diet, Clarkson was able to identify and eliminate problematic foods, resulting in significant weight loss and better general health.

The Plant Paradox diet focuses on full, nutrient-dense foods while restricting or eliminating lectin-rich foods such as beans, grains, and nightshades. Clarkson discovered that by making these basic improvements, she was able to:

- Reduce inflammation and bloating

- Boost her energy levels

- Improve her overall well-being

Clarkson shed an astonishing 40 pounds in a year, but more importantly, she experienced substantial changes in her health and vitality. Even during the COVID-19 pandemic, she maintained her healthy practices, demonstrating the need of consistency and self-care in long-term success.

Clarkson's journey has motivated many people to take care of their own health. Her success story also serves as a reminder that losing weight is about more than just the number on the scale; it's also about developing a stronger relationship with our bodies and thoughts. We, too, can achieve transformative weight reduction journeys by focusing on nourishment, self-care, and sustainability, as Kelly Clarkson has.

Clarkson discussed her journey on several shows and social media, describing how she attempted to improve her overall health after being diagnosed with a thyroid problem and an autoimmune disease.

Clarkson's diet emphasized whole foods, lean proteins, and healthy oils while avoiding processed and sugary foods, gluten, and soy. She also included exercise and stress management techniques in her routine. Her attitude was not only about losing weight but also about improving her entire health and treating her thyroid condition.

It's amazing to see Clarkson putting her health first and sharing her experience with her fans!

CONCLUSION

As we come to the end of THE PLANT PARADOX LIFESTYLE: 18 Steps to Help You Lose Weight, Reduce Chronic Inflammation, Heal Your Gut, and Rapidly Improve Your Health, it becomes evident that real change is about adopting a new way of life rather than merely adhering to a set of guidelines.

These 18 steps are intended to lead you on a path to greater health, where each decision you make brings you one step closer to living a full, active, and healthy life. Whether it's reconsidering your eating philosophy, understanding the value of fasting, or discovering delight in the art of cooking, each step brings you closer to becoming the best version of yourself.

This way of living focuses on internal healing, reducing chronic inflammation, and promoting gut health in addition to weight loss. Recall that transformation is an ongoing process.

By embracing the ideas presented in this book, you're making a commitment to a lifetime of wellness rather than merely sticking to a diet. Let Kelly Clarkson's achievement serve as motivation for you as you follow these steps, understanding that true, long-lasting improvement is attainable.

FAQs

1. What is the Plant Paradox program? The Plant Paradox program is a dietary and lifestyle plan developed by Dr. Steven Gundry that focuses on eliminating lectins—proteins found in certain plants—that can cause inflammation and other health issues.

2. Why should I stay away from lectins, and what are they? Lectins are proteins found in various foods, including grains, beans, and certain vegetables. For some people, lectins can contribute to inflammation, digestive issues, and other health problems.

3. Is the Plant Paradox program suitable for everyone? While many people benefit from the Plant Paradox program, it's important to consult with a healthcare professional before making any significant dietary changes, especially if you have existing health conditions.

4. Can I still eat out while following the Plant Paradox program? Yes, you can eat out while following the Plant Paradox program. It's important to make informed choices and ask about ingredients, but many restaurants offer options that align with the program's guidelines.

5. How long does it take to see results on the Plant Paradox program? The timeline for seeing results varies from person to person, but many people notice improvements in their health within a few weeks of starting the program.

ACKNOWLEDGMENT

I would like to express my sincere gratitude to everyone who helped me all through the journey when I was writing this book. Your support and guidance have helped me. To my readers, I appreciate the time you took to read these pages. I hope your road toward wellness is fruitful and fulfilling. Please consider leaving a review if you find this book to be helpful; it may benefit others who are looking for similar information.

ABOUT THE AUTHOR

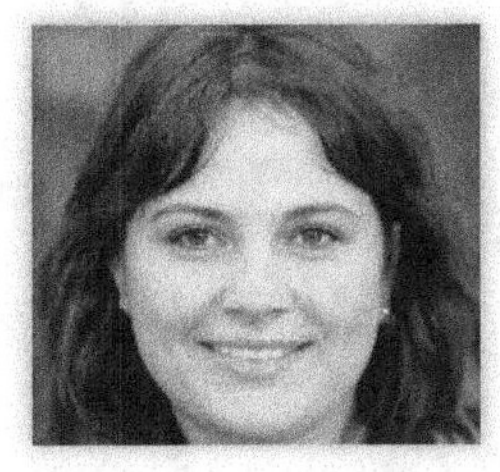 Nathalie Smith is a passionate health and wellness advocate who strives to help others improve their health via informed lifestyle choices. Nathalie has obtained vital insights on the importance of diet, nutrition, and mindful living through a personal journey that began with an exploration of various health theories and practices. Her experiences have inspired her to adopt and advocate the concepts contained in "The Plant Paradox Lifestyle," which she discusses in her book. Nathalie's goal is to use her own experiences, both triumphs and setbacks to encourage and mentor others as they pursue their paths toward optimal health.